Vegan Diet:

How to Live a Healthier Lifestyle, Lose Weight, and Experience Limitless Energy Levels through the Vegan Diet

Kendra R. Davis

Table of Contents

Introduction

Are you trying all sorts of diets and realizing nothing is working? Is it hard to keep up with the energy of others? Are you tired of looking in the mirror and not liking what you see? If you answered yes to these questions, look no further. The answer is simple: a vegan diet. Yes, a diet free of animal products, including milk and cheese, is the easiest way to lose weight, be healthy, feel more energized, and save the Earth while you're at it.

Now, I know exactly what must be going through your head right now. "Why would I ever give up meat and dairy? That is way too extreme!" There are more questions popping in your head, such as protein deficiency, vitamin deficiency, what do vegans even eat, and much more. It's understandable. A vegan diet is a mystery to many people, and to others it seems like a joke.

Don't worry; all of these questions will be answered. It may be hard to envision yourself on a vegan diet, but it is the best possible thing you can do for your body. In just a month you will feel the difference and you will be thanking yourself for making the switch. In a few years, when you realize what a positive impact your diet change has had on your life, it will be an even happier day. Do yourself a favor and start treating your body right today. By reading this, you will understand why you should go vegan, get answers to the questions you may have, and finally, learn how to make the change.

The Protein Debacle: Despite what is Believed, Vegans Can Get Plenty of Protein

Probably the question a vegan gets asked most is: "But where do you get your protein?"

Well, to be honest, America is obsessed with protein intake. It is more likely to suffer side effects from too much protein than too little. If you are consuming a healthy vegan diet, full of legumes, leafy greens, quinoa, tofu, and other things, you will get enough protein to fuel an army! Many vegan athletes are challenging the stereotype of athletes needing meat and dairy to build muscle with the plentiful sources of protein. Being vegan is normally associated with a skinny girl who hasn't bathed in a couple of weeks to conserve water.

The truth is, vegans are everywhere! And they aren't all skinny girls. Carrie Underwood is vegan, and we all know how great those legs are. Natalie Portman, Mike Tyson (it's true—I swear!), Ellen DeGeneres, Usher, and many other celebrities are vegan. Jennifer Lopez even went vegan for a while in order to lose 10 pounds and get back on track. Back to Mike Tyson, he lost 100 points and flushed all the drugs out of his system with a simple diet change.

Yes—it is absolutely possible to get plenty of protein and other nutrients needed in a vegan diet. Actually, it is more likely that you will receive more nutrients because you are eating foods filled with nutrients and vitamins! Assuming that you are eating a healthy vegan diet and not shelling out money on frozen vegan pizzas and fake meat. Those are obviously healthier than real pizzas and meat and are delicious on certain occasions, but they should still be eaten sparingly. You don't want to go vegan just to become a "junk-food vegan" munching on Oreos (yep, Oreos are vegan) and fake cheese!

Protein is one of America's main obsessions that really doesn't have the science to back it up. Science says Americans, on average, take in twice the amount of protein than necessary. People do not need that much protein. It is more than possible to overdose on protein, and probably more likely than not getting enough protein. Overdosing can lead to kidney disease and cancer, and other things that are bad for you! Too much protein involves more nitrogen than needed, which hurts the kidneys.

If you are really looking to lose weight while doing the cruelty free diet, it is important to be a healthy vegan and to get the nutrients you need. The only vitamin that a vegan is maybe missing is vitamin B12, but luckily there are plenty of supplements out there, some which are liquid and you take a shot of it in order to get it in your system, or you can just have a pill. Also, there are some cereals, some brands of nutritional yeast (which is the vegan form of cheese and oh so yummy), and some soymilk has B12 in it. The word you can look for is cyanocobalamin, which is vitamin B12, and the absolute best form of it. Otherwise, all of the nutrients are covered in a healthy vegan diet, full of vegetables, fruit, grains, and legumes.

So, where do vegans get their protein? From plenty of places, and it's more than likely that they are getting closer to the recommended amount than a meat-eater would be.

The Scare-Tactic: The Damaging Ways of the Meat Industry

If you are one of those people that gets offended easily by people telling you what you are doing is wrong, you might as well skip this chapter right now. Seriously. Don't read it. It will only make you defensive because your eyes will be opened and then you will be mad because you'll wish that you could just close them again.

For those brave enough to read on, imagine walking through a barn full of chickens stuffed into cages, fed growth hormones and popping out eggs more than they should be. It smells. It's gross. It's inhumane. The chickens are in cages with less than an inch of foot-room. Some are dead in their cages, others are seriously ill. This is most likely how that chicken you had for lunch was raised. Less than an inch of room it's entire life. Stuffed with growth hormones, and maybe living next to a dead chicken it's entire life. Or maybe it was the dead chicken's leg that you just ate. Oh, you're buying "free range" chickens? It's still more than likely that these chickens were raised in an inhumane way. They still are transported to the same slaughterhouses and burned and mutilated while they are still conscious.

Animals are smart. Pigs are smart enough to indicate temperature preferences, play simple games, and to let you know if they like you or not, and remember it. That's why when they are poked, prodded, shocked, dragged across rooms and cut open for food, it can seem like murder to those who work there. Some people are actually scarred and have mental problems after working in an animal farm for a while.

I'm not trying to gross you into eating vegan, I'm just saying that the animals you eat on a daily basis (assuming you're eating meat) aren't treated as you would like to think. They don't get a chance to live life, frolic through fields, and receive any attention or love. This isn't the movie Babe. These animals that are raised for food are stuffed with hormones and chemicals so they grow faster so they can get killed faster and turn into to that "delicious burger" from McDonalds. Also, if they are stuffed with growth hormones and chemicals to make them grow faster and you are eating the meat that comes from these animals, imagine what you are ingesting. Chemicals, hormones, and other nasty stuff that is in the meat of the animals because they were eating it is all going into your body through that "wonderful" steak. Every single thing you put in your mouth affects the composition of your body. Same goes for animals. So that meat still has growth hormones and nasty chemicals in it, and you're putting it in your mouth. Gross, right? Wouldn't you rather put organic fruits and vegetables in your body and have the luxury of knowing that it was grown naturally and in a cruelty-free way, without ingesting any nasty chemicals that aren't made to go into human bodies?

If that doesn't get to you, maybe this will. Animals raised like this have more of a negative impact on the environment than humans do. The United States alone could literally feed almost a billion people with the grains that the cows and other animals eat that we raise for meat. Imagine, if we didn't have these cows that we are stuffing to grow fast enough to kill, we would all be rolling in the grains. Enough to share with a few countries, at least. Not to mention the gases these cows let out after they finish consuming these grains are toxic to the atmosphere. The animal farming industry is harmful to the soil, is taking up lands, is polluting water, and polluting air. So, one could say that by eating meat, you are directly contributing to damage to the environment.

Plus, meat has so many contaminants in it besides chemicals, included feces, blood, and other fluids. Many types of chicken contain traces of a dangerous bacterium that is the direct source of food poisoning. We all know how a bout of food poisoning feels, with cramping, pain, diarrhea, vomiting, fever, and other terrible things. Let's try to avoid that by not eating meat!

Okay, that's the end of my scare tactic. I think you get it by now. There's a lot more I could tell you about the inhumane practices of the meat industry, but I think the bare basics are covered. Every person that goes vegan saves over 100 animals a year. If that doesn't make you proud, what could?

The Easiest Way to Lose Weight For Good

As we've discussed, there is an easy way to lose weight, and it's all in the vegan diet. No meat, no growth hormones, and no dairy. You understand why you should give up meat after this last chapter, but why exactly do you need to cut out dairy? Well, that's a good question.

Let's think about what milk is used for. We drink it when we are babies in order to grow. Why would we ever want to drink a large animal's baby-growing substance? Sure, it tastes good, but there are so many alternatives that it isn't made to grow a baby cow into a huge adult cow. The milk that is taken from cows is made for the babies, not for human consumption.

Cows are also not treated as well as we would like them to be. Some farms will milk the cows until they bleed. Cows aren't meant to produce milk for the demands of all humans. They are over-milked and it hurts them. Not to mention there are probably traces of blood in your morning glass of milk or coffee creamer.

Now, I bet you are thinking about how milk gives us calcium and we need that in order to keep our bones healthy. Calcium comes in many different forms, and there is honestly no evidence to show that milk is a significant source of calcium for our bodies. Milk actually has the reverse effect than strengthening our bones. It is an acidic animal protein. Once it is in our bodies, our body fights it to make sure it doesn't damage anything and it gives up the density of our bones. Studies have actually shown that drinking milk is linked to more fractures in people because of bone density depletion. Put that glass of milk down right now and pick up some soy or nut-based milk. It tastes just as good and is way better for your precious body.

Still worried about calcium? Go ahead and eat white beans, sardines, dried figs, bok choy, kale, black-eyed peas, almonds, oranges, turnip greens, sesame seeds, broccoli, seaweed, and tofu. There are plenty of options besides calf growing cow milk, and some are actually better options for calcium than milk. Plus, if we drink milk, the calcium isn't absorbed as well as the vegan calcium is. Protein causes calcium loss through urine, along with too much sodium, smoking and caffeine. Give up those vices now ladies, and keep that calcium in your system! Instead of doing that, you can exercise, go outside and absorb that vitamin D, and eat your veggies and fruits!

Cheese is the same way, as it is made from milk. It is fattening, simply put. Ten pounds of milk makes one pound of cheese, on average. It is heated up and bacteria are added, along with an enzyme that makes milk "clot." Then, it becomes a gel and is cooked until it is at the texture that they want, and then drained. Then, it is handled, salted, and pressed. After that it is cured and aged for a minimum of 60 days, because otherwise it wouldn't be safe to eat. We already talked about how bad milk is for you, imagine eating it in condensed form! So much worse for you. Also, why would you want to put heated milk that has bacteria added in your body? Sure, it might be considered "good" bacteria, but it still sounds gross and unnatural.

Humans aren't really made to digest that, either. Ever wonder why some people are lactose intolerant and simply can't handle milk products? That might have something to do with it. Yes, cheese is absolutely delicious. But there are plenty of vegan-friendly cheese options nowadays that can even melt on homemade pizzas or grilled cheeses. It won't taste the exact same at first, but your body will be thanking you big time. Go buy some fake cheese and kick out the real kind. Nutritional yeast also creates a cheesy flavor to a lot of things.

Let's move on to eggs. So healthy for you and what-not, according to the world. Have you ever thought about what an egg actually is? Eggs are unfertilized chickens, which means it is literally a chicken period. Let me repeat that: a chicken period. And we all want to cook it and eat it for breakfast and put it in our baked goods. It is honestly disgusting!

The cholesterol levels in eggs are off the charts, and are actually comparable to a hamburger! That can increase your cholesterol level and lead to cardiovascular disease. Also, have you ever heard of salmonella poisoning? Eggs poison over 100,000 Americans each year. Okay, so you think you'll buy organic to try to avoid that. Wrong. Still has the same levels of cholesterol, the same negative effects on your body, and still really does not help the chicken out.

Standard egg companies throw out any male chicken, either just killing them or grinding them up (most of the time alive) to make meat. Why? Male chickens are not nearly as profitable as female chickens because it takes more to raise them than they would get from profit. Females, on the other hand, are good for eggs and they are good for meat later on. The standard companies need the eggs as quickly as they can possibly get them, so, they take the chicken and let it starve for a couple of days until the body goes into egg-making mode. Not to mention, these poor birds are stuffed in such small cages that they probably never get a chance to even spread one wing.

Sure, scrambled eggs taste good in the morning, but next time you are craving that, maybe try scrambled tofu instead. Better for the environment and your cholesterol levels, not to mention the chicken.

While we are talking about giving up dairy products, I will tell you that it is the easiest possible way to drop weight fast. Give up the dairy, and literally watch the weight fall off your body. Plus, you'll feel like a million bucks!

What else do you need to do to get that rocking bod? I'm going to say something that may make you drop this book right now and say "No way! You're crazy!" People, we've got to stop putting alcohol in our body. Yep, I said it. Quit drinking. Okay, now altogether that might be impossible, so it is acceptable once in a while, just like eating sugary foods is acceptable once in a while, but we have to stop doing it every night or every weekend. Yes, there are some good health benefits for having a small glass of wine each night, but the negatives far outweigh the positives. First of all, alcohol is filled with calories. One beer is over 200 calories, and wine isn't much better. Alcohol has no nutritional value whatsoever, so its basically drinking calories that provide nothing to your body but drunkenness and a loss of senses. So try not to get wasted as often. If you don't drink much already, good for you! Keep up the good work. I know it's a hard habit to break, as it can really help relax you after a long day, but maybe try some teas instead. There are natural herbs out there that can relax you like no other.

While I'm on this roll of what you should kick out of your body, lets talk about some more things.

- **Sugar:** It's bad for you, highly addictive, and a leading contributor to diabetes and obesity. It also has a ton of cholesterol in it as well and may give you heart disease. Not to mention it is bad for your teeth and is completely empty calories, with no added nutrition. Stevia is a much better alternative for you.

- **Artificial Flavoring:** It's made in a lab from chemicals that do not have any health benefits and it has some sort of detrimental effect on your health.

- **Enriched wheat:** Key nutrients are stripped out while the wheat is refined, and then niacin, thiamine, riboflavin, folic acid, and iron are added after they nutrients are stripped. Not enough to make it actually healthy for you, though.

- **Hydrogenated (Fractionated) Oils:** These are oils that have been heated and then cooled quickly, which essentially takes out the liquid, leaving a large amount of fat. Before they were processed, they were probably very healthy, but now they are processed and completely unhealthy. Do not buy anything with this on the list.

- **High fructose corn syrup:** This is so terrible for you and your body. It may also be under the name corn sugar. It is lethal for you, causing hypertension, diabetes, weight gain (which if you're reading this, you probably want to avoid this like the plague), and much more. Watch for it in fruit juices especially.

- **Artificial coloring:** Why would you want to eat something that has been dyed? I'll just leave it at that.

- **Aspartame and Sucralose:** Fake sugars are not healthier than actual sugars. These have deadly ingredients in them and you do not want to put it in your body. The brand names it would be under are Splenda, NutraSweet, and Equal. Check protein shakes, too!

- **MSG:** Also known as natural flavoring, yeast extract, autolyzed yeast extract, textured protein, etc. Basically, this is modified, has no nutrients, vitamins or minerals, and can give you migraines, obesity, ALS, Parkinson's, and other types of terrible things. Avoid this one for sure.

- **Canola oil:** This oil is poisonous, and works great as insect repellant. To eat? Not so great.
- **Soy Lecithin:** Essential, this is a waste product, and contains pesticides and it comes in the form of basically sludge. Do not put sludge in your body!

Basically, the summary of this chapter is to read your labels. If you don't understand what something is, or you see something that is unhealthy for you like high fructose corn syrup, put it down and walk away. We want to be healthy, and it is almost impossible to be healthy if you are putting things into your body that you don't even know what they are!

It's okay to indulge sometimes of course, and I know this is a lot coming at you at once. We will cover how to tackle changing your diet in a different chapter. It's scary, but just imagine how great you'll feel. Don't picture it as "giving up" these items, really think of it as taking over your body and deciding what to put in it for yourself.

Aren't Humans Meant to Eat Meat Because We Are Superior?

This is another question that tops the charts on veganism. Aren't animals there for us to eat and consume? We are the superior beings in this situation, and we can hunt them. Animals eat other animals, why isn't it okay for humans to eat them?

This is yet another a good question, but when you think about it, animals eat other animals because they can hunt them down. Think of an animal that is a predator. For example, a lion. It runs down its prey and claws at it, bites it, and ultimately kills it with no help. What do humans need to kill an animal? A weapon. We can't chase down an animal in the wilderness and kill it with our bare hands. We need help with killing animals. For example, we use guns, arrows, spears, something to help us kill. We don't have the necessary equipment on our bodies in order to hunt successfully; we have to use a helping tool.

Now, we may be superior with technology, sure, but there's no possible way we would be able to hunt like an animal that is built to hunt. Animals hunt each other to keep nature's numbers in check. It is part of the food chain and it is part of life. We are at the top of the food chain. Yes we can eat animals if we want to because of weapons and technology. But that doesn't mean that we should. Nature doesn't intend for us to eat animals just because we can create weapons and hunt animals down with them.

Even if we could hunt down animals and catch them, we still have to cook them before we eat it. The animals that hunt do not have to build a fire and roast the meat over it; they rip into it and eat it raw. Even when we do cook and eat meat, our bodies still aren't made to digesting meat.

We are made to eat plants, from our teeth to our digestive tract. Our teeth are flat and made to chew plants, much like the plant-eating animals. When you look at the teeth of a lion or a dog, they are sharp and made to rip into flesh. Our teeth are made to grind down plants. Our hands are made to gather plants and vegetables, not to claw our way through skin and flesh.

Animals have a stomach with high acidity in the juices, which will break down the meat in the stomach. Our digestive tract would be similar to that of herbivores. Our saliva starts the process and we have a long intestinal tract in order to digest plants. Meat-eating animals have shorter tracts, which are ideal for digesting meat.

So, in short, no. It is not "natural" for humans to eat meat. In fact, because we are the superior beings, we should be in charge of looking out for the animals, not mass-producing them in terrible conditions for our gratification.

Fight the Diseases and Eat Your Greens!

Not only are vegans generally slimmer, they are also quite a bit healthier naturally too. Vegans have a much lower chance of cardiovascular disease, which kills about 1 million Americans per year. Why? Because vegans do not consumer animal fat or cholesterol and do consume more fiber and nutrient-dense fruits and vegetables.

Seventy percent of diseases are related to diet. So, when you clean up your diet and cut out unhealthy foods, it is no mystery that you are avoiding these. To those people consuming questionable ingredients and who knows what from meat, they might be putting themselves at risk.

Now I'm not saying that if you go vegan, you'll never get sick. I'm just saying you have a much better chance of fighting off diseases and preventing them, especially the mega bad ones.

Vegans and vegetarians add on about 13 healthy years to your life. That is a ton of time! That is like being born and going all the way to 8th grade again, which is a lot of time. If you don't want an extra thirteen years on your life to watch your kids have kids and be retired and have fun, go ahead and keep shoveling that meat in your mouth.

Back to food poisoning, the CDC says that about 76 million people get food poisoning each year, resulting in over three hundred thousand hospitalizations and about five thousand deaths. Meat is way more likely to be involved in creating these than any fruits or vegetables.

Not to mention avoiding diseases, you'll also have a lot more energy by eating a plant-based diet. Too much fat clogs the arteries and doesn't give your muscles enough oxygen. This makes a person feel extremely tired and exhausted. When you eat a plant-based diet, you get plenty of nutrients while still feeling satisfied in the stomach. You'll be amazed at how much energy you feel while eating plants. If you kick out caffeine (which, you don't have to, but it will make you more energized) and have a glass of fresh fruit juice, you'll feel like you've never felt before. You'll be totally energized and ready for the day. It's amazing how much easier you can keep up with things when you aren't feeling bogged down by unhealthy meats and dairy products slugging through your system.

Ever heard the saying that the more color on your plate the better? It's true. The reason fruits and vegetables are colored is because of the phytochemicals that are in them, which fight diseases. The more colorful your plate is, the better. It fills your body with great nutrients and strengthens your immune system. Produce is one of the best things you can fill your body with. Veggie plates and fruit plates should be your new best friend. They fill you up, make you healthy, and do all of that without even adding too many calories to your count.

Not only does all of this happen, but a healthy heart happens too. Vegans have lower cholesterol and have a lot less chance of heart disease. We also have lower blood pressure. It has actually been proven that people with high blood pressure who start a vegan diet do not need medicine after their diet change.

Worried about diabetes? No need to worry. If you eat a healthy vegan diet, full of complex carbohydrates and fiber, low in fat and low in sugar, too, it can reduce the need for medicine, or even take it completely away. Eating a diet like that is easy if you eat what we have been talking about! And finally, cancer is also prevented. You reduce your risk by at least half if you eat a vegan diet!

So, in short, a vegan diet is so much healthier for you, and helps your body become strong so that it can fight diseases and ultimately, you can live a longer, healthier life. Eat your greens, yellows, purples, oranges, and reds in order to fight diseases and be healthier than you can imagine ever being. It is super simple to feel healthy with a simple diet change!

Are you ready to change your life by eating compassionately? Don't worry, it doesn't have to be a cold turkey, give up everything at once type deal. We will cover how to tackle this huge lifestyle change in the next section, and it will be surprisingly easier than you think!

So, You Want To Be a Vegan

I hope that you have decided to make the switch, or at least give it a try. I challenge you, even if you are thinking that this is still way too extreme for you, to try it for at least a month. Just a month! If you don't feel completely better, full of energy, and happier, well, you can chuck this book and never read it again. But I promise you that you will feel like a completely different person! Not only will you have more energy and feel better about what your putting in your mouth, but you will also lose weight like you never have before. Cutting out meat and dairy is a surefire way to drop a few pounds pretty much instantly.

Okay, so thirty days, right? It will be hard at first, I'm not saying it's going to be easy breezy to give it all up and treat your body better. It will feel extremely hard, and some days you'll want to stuff your face with everything unhealthy you can find, especially during certain times of the month (sorry to any guys reading this, but it's true). Some days you just want to be super unhealthy, and its okay because you can still eat unhealthy vegan noms. With the demand for vegan items on the rise, there are more and more options out there, ranging from vegan cookies to vegan ice cream, and even some vegan frozen pizzas. You'll still have plenty of junk food options, no worries.

I don't want you to feel like this is impossible, and I also don't want you to think negatively about this. It may seem hard, but it is totally possible, even if you are used to living on meat and dairy and practically nothing else. Don't think of it as if you are giving up everything; think about what you can eat instead. You'll be surprised at the results that come up if you do a web search for vegan recipes. A lot of it is the stuff you know and love, and you can adapt them to your taste buds and make them awesome.

There are a few different ways you can dive into transitioning your lifestyle into this healthier, happier way of living. Lets cover those now.

Method One: Cold Turkey

You're determined, ready and you want to get it done right now. Now that your eyes are open, the idea of meat and dairy disgusts you and you'd rather never touch it again. Does this describe you? Awesome! I'm glad you're ready to get started. You seem really determined, and that is very admirable. Good for you. Go cold turkey. Go through the fridge and pantry and get rid of everything that doesn't fit the new lifestyle. Go grocery shopping, read labels, and stick to what you know. You've got this and you're going for it. Stick to the produce area and pick out organic fruits and vegetable and other items.

This might be the bravest option of all, but it is very admirable. You understand that eating meat is harmful to the environment, animals, and most importantly, your body and you won't stand for it anymore. You are in control of what goes into your body and even though you can eat whatever you want, you will only choose the healthiest options. You realize it might be hard for a while. It might feel like you're missing out when you politely decline that piece of decadent cheesecake when you're out to dinner, or have to ask for a salad with no cheese, croutons, or dairy based dressing. In the long run, though, you know it is best for your body. You will feel amazing, look amazing, and the self-control you are practicing in your diet will go to other parts of your life. Taking control of your diet is the first step to becoming, well, quite frankly, awesome. If you can do this, and just start it out cold turkey, imagine what else you can do! You are a powerful person, and you've got this. There's even a phone app that will give you plenty of starting recipes. It's called the 21-Day Vegan Kick Start and it is a free app! Check it out!

Method Two: Baby Steps

It's okay if you aren't quite ready to tackle method one. It's a hard habit to break, eating unhealthy. Actually, it's addicting to eat unhealthy, which is why we keep doing it even when we feel awful afterwards. So, if you aren't quite ready to give it all up, give up one thing at a time. First, you can start with red meats. They might be the nastiest of all. After a week or two of eating no red meat, add something else on that you need to give up. Start with things you might think will be easier for you! Then, each week you can celebrate your successes and add more and more until you are eating at your satisfaction. This is probably the easiest way to transition, because as you go on, you will find it easier because you'll be feeling healthier and better about life. You'll realize you don't need the things that you used to eat, and you're just as happy with a kick-butt salad for lunch in place of the burger you used to eat daily.

Baby steps are all it takes to get to an amazing body, higher energy levels, and an overall feeling of healthfulness. Always keep the goal in mind, keep the body you want pictured, and keep taking steps to get there. Seems easy enough, right? You don't have to do it all at once; you just have to keep moving towards your goal, like in other areas of life.

Another way of doing the baby step method is to go vegan on Monday. Just Monday. One day a week, eat the vegan diet. Then, after you're used to that, up it to two days a week, and so on. This method will give you a taste of what its like one day a week, and you'll be able to slowly transition to doing it more and more, until finally you're all the way to the healthiest diet of your life!

Notice how you feel when you eat vegan compared to when you eat normally. More than likely, you'll feel lighter, less bloated, and just generally better. It is amazing how your diet affects the way you feel each day. The baby step method will magnify this feeling because you will go from one day eating clean, to the next day eating meat. Notice the changes. Then, you'll know you're doing the right thing.

Method Three: Detox

Detoxing is always a good way to start a new lifestyle, but it can be very challenging. For a long, long time, humans have used fasting and detoxing as a way to connect with their bodies and lose weight. It is important to do the detox correctly, however. It is transitioned into slowly, by each day eating more and more healthy. Then, once you are on the detox, you can follow the rules of the detox. Some are liquid only, maybe fresh fruit and vegetable juices or smoothies, or even soup broth. Others allow only raw fruits and vegetables. The most intense kind is water only.

Detoxing should only last 3-10 days. Any longer than this, and your body will be in starvation mode. It is to cleanse yourself and rid yourself of toxins from the nasty food you've been eating, not to starve yourself.

During a detox, you may experience headaches, nausea, dizziness, and other symptoms. That is your body getting rid of the toxins and taking it out of you. You'll be extremely hungry for a few days, but then at a certain point, you will feel light and happy. You will be toxin free, and then you will slowly re-introduce food back into your system. It's important not to go from 0 to 100 with these, you need to introduce raw vegetables back in and then slowly add more each meal.

Detoxing is not for everyone, but it can definitely cleanse the system and feel great. Doctors now are saying that there is no proof that it works, but people have been doing it for literally thousands of years. Fasting is even in the Bible! It's been around for quite a while, and it is a common practice to focus on things and to lose weight and connect with your body. The power of that is amazing, although it takes a ton of self-control, and is very difficult to achieve.

Beyoncé fasted for one of her roles in a movie, called Dream Girls. She lost 20 pounds by fasting and only consuming liquids. Fasting is not a long-term option, though, you only want to do it for a couple of days or there can be negative health effects. There are many debates out there about if fasting is good for you or not. Some people say that it has a negative effect on metabolism and can raise risks. Others will swear that it can regenerate the body and even the immune system. So, what side should you be on? I say you decide for yourself. Give it a try, see how it feels, if you hate it, and then introduce food back into your diet sooner. Simple.

After a detox, especially if you are doing it from a meat eating diet, you will notice you have lost weight, but it is absolutely vital to change your diet to something healthier after the detox, or you will just gain it right back. No one wants to go through all that for nothing, right? After your detox, slowly introduce healthy foods back into your body, and stick with healthy foods. We want to look and feel amazing, and the only way to do that is to eat foods that are amazing for you. It's pointless to do a detox if you're just going to eat the same crap you did before. Don't waste it!

Those are the three methods I suggest. There certainly are other methods, but those are the simplest and most effective ways to do it. On all three methods, another important thing is to not dive right in to only eating the vegan substitutes for meat. Don't replace your favorite food with fake favorite food, because it won't taste the same and it will only frustrate you. Find new options and new things you love, and then down the road a bit, when you try that vegan burger, it will taste amazing. You need to expand your horizons. Soon, you'll realize how much you can eat and what you can do with vegetables and fruits and the possibilities will seem endless.

Whatever you do, don't come up with excuses on why you are going to wait. So it will be hard? Nothing in life worth having is easy. You really want to push off feeling better and looking better? Why? Just do it. Take steps towards it and do it. If, after thirty days, you are cursing this book and everything to do with it, you don't feel better, and you haven't lost weight, by all means, eat meat again. Do whatever you want. Just try it, though, and try it now.

Money, Money, Money

Many people say that vegan diets are more expensive. Is that true? It can be. Fake meat will range from 3-7 dollars a little package. Dairy-free ice cream can get to be a little pricy. Dairy-free yogurt is almost double regular yogurt. So, yes, it can be more expensive if you're indulging in all of these things. If you are eating fruits and vegetables, and other healthy items, it can be a lot cheaper than a regular diet. But think about how much money you are spending on meat, anyway. Normally a pound of meat is 3-10 dollars, on average, and can be even more. If you don't buy meat, you can save money in the long run.

Plus, you're avoiding diseases, so you're actually saving money in comparison to eating meat. You won't have to spend as much money on doctor bills or medicine. You'll feel better and more energetic, so you won't spend as much on morning coffee or energy drinks. You should, instead, put money towards joining a gym and working out regularly. Then, you'll sleep better and look better, if you use your gym membership. Working out has so many benefits to it as well, imagine how much good you'll be doing for yourself if you work out and eat a healthy vegan diet!

Speaking of a healthy vegan diet, spend the extra money on organic produce when you can. This money is going straight towards your health! You need to treat yourself. Why spend extra money on a handbag that you could spend insuring that you are getting naturally grown produce and no extra chemicals in your body? This is your body. This is what enables you to do the activities you do every day. Don't skimp out on yourself. You need to be healthy, and you deserve to be healthy. Spend the extra money.

If a lot of people go vegan and buy produce and the vegan fake-meats, think about how the stores will be forced to carry more in order to support the demand. Money talks! If we start spending out money on healthier items, we can basically use our money to speak to the companies that we need more. One of the recent big successes of money talking is at Dunkin Doughnuts. They recently started making vegan coffees available, made with almond milk. If that isn't money talking, I'm not sure what is. They saw the demand, and they seized the opportunity. Now, we are just waiting for them to formulate a vegan doughnut! If that day ever comes, I'm sure there will be a lot of happy vegans. (Don't worry; you can still make your own doughnuts if you're obsessed).

So, money talks. Why do you think a vegan saves over 100 animals a year? Because there is less demand for the meat that they used to eat, and therefore, they don't have to murder as many animals in order to meet the demand of the crowd. If we all stopped buying meat, they wouldn't have to murder any animals. But, that is far off, although maybe someday it will happen! If even 10 people who read this book decide to go vegan, that's 1,000 animals saved. The difference you can make with your money and your diet is amazing. It is the most powerful tool you have. So use it! Use your money to talk to corporations and use your diet to talk to other people.

People will look at you and wonder what is different about you. Maybe they'll ask you about it, and you can share with them what you have learned. Try not to sound too preachy or anything; that is a total turnoff to people. Just explain what you've learned and why you decided to try it. Do not ever tell anyone to change if they don't want to hear it. Sure, this book is filled with me telling you why you need to change, but I didn't shove it into your hands, you picked it up. Obviously, you were a little curious to begin with and you wanted to know, so here is everything you need to know in this book. However, if you decide to run around town telling everyone at restaurants to put the meat down, it probably won't go over well. Laid-back vegans are the best vegans. People will notice no matter what you do, so don't push it onto people!

So, basically, spend your money in the right places, and soon they will stop killing animals, and the places that manufacture vegan meats will have a higher demand and make more yummy "meats" for us to eat! Eat right and people will notice, but don't force it upon them. Let it happen naturally. Even if someone decides to give up red meat because of what they see in you, that's a step in the right direction and you should be proud that you made that difference!

Time for a Change: Buying Vegan Goods

So, you're ready to dive in, but you have no idea where to start. That's okay! Everyone starts in different places. In general, vegan goods should be at pretty much any grocery store. It might be in the healthy "organic" section of the grocery store, or it could just be stuck in with the rest of the goods. A general rule of thumb is that tofu and some vegan meats are often found in the produce section, kind of around the place where those specialty dressings are, and next to the lettuce. I've always found tofu and vegan cheeses around there, along with some vegan hot dogs and tofurkey.

Next, the frozen section is your new best friend. Frozen fruits and veggies are a lifesaver when you're in a pinch and not sure what to cook. Also, there will be the fake meats in the frozen section. They could be by the fruits and veggies, but they also tend to be hanging around in the "single dinners" section. You'll see a bunch labeled "Morning Star" or "Gardein." Personal favorite brand is Gardein. Everything they make is 100% vegan and so delicious. They make beef and chicken sliders, chicken tenders, mandarin chicken, meatballs, and so much more. You don't even have to read the ingredients if its that brand, because everything is vegan. Amy's is another good brand, making organic and delicious meals you can warm up for a quick meal. It's important to read the ingredients in that, though, because some still contain eggs, cheese and milk. The same goes for Morning Star and Boca brand foods. Their lines are really good and very tasty, but unfortunately, many of them still contain dairy products. After what we have learned about dairy products, let's try not to consume those even if the fake meat is delicious that comes from it.

Besides those, there's nutritional yeast that is pretty much a staple in a vegan diet. You can add it to anything to make it taste cheesy. There's even recipes for vegan cheese-its that use this magic powder. This can be found in health food stores, or, if you live in a small town, you can actually order it online and it will not perish while shipping to you. TVP is another amazing thing, which is short for textured vegetable protein. Super easy to make, and it will taste like beef if prepared and spiced properly. It may take you a few tries, but soon it will be easy.

Next, there's the tofu and the tempeh. Both are tricky to prepare. Tempeh is probably easier, but it has a nutty taste if it isn't marinated long enough. Tofu is very versatile and contains a lot of protein. It does need to be pressed if you are planning to use it like meat. Put paper towels under and over it, put something heavy on top of it, and then wait 30 minutes to an hour before you try to cook with it. This will give it a firm texture and it will cook better. Another option is freezing it, which will firm it even more. Do your research and play around with it. You'll get it down soon enough! There's also an app by the tofu brand Nasoya that has compiled recipes on it, called All Things Tofu. It's free, so feel free to go check it out if you have a smart phone.

The easiest way to learn about vegan foods is to get a few vegan cookbooks and look through them. You'll learn so much it will amaze you. Or, just go online and do a quick web search. You'll learn more with each meal you cook, and you'll get better at preparing foods.

Are you worried more about going out to eat and being the weird person who can't order anything? Many restaurants are used to accommodating people, and there is absolutely nothing wrong with calling ahead or looking online at the menu before you go. Sometimes, you may end up with a pathetic looking side salad with no dressing, but that's okay, because you can always eat when you get home. Many restaurants are getting a lot better at accommodating vegans because they are becoming more prevalent everywhere. There are also many restaurants that specialize in vegan and vegetarian foods, but those tend to be in larger cities. There are a lot more options than you originally thought. There are also apps for your phone that will help you find a vegan restaurant or at least a vegan restaurant nearby. The app HappyCow helps you find health stores and vegan-friendly restaurant.

You don't have to do this alone. There are plenty of others taking this journey, and you'll be surprised at who supports your new healthy journey.

Prepare Yourself for the Questions

Now that you've gone vegan, you are likely to get a lot of questions. I've already debunked some of them, including where do you get your protein, and aren't humans made to eat meat? But there will be so many more questions. Why are you doing this? Isn't it hard?

Then come the jokes. Being a vegan at a Thanksgiving Dinner might be a challenge that no one can ever prepare for. If your family is anything like mine, every year, they will ask you if you want some turkey. Every year, you will politely decline and they will laugh and laugh and the quiz you more on why you don't eat meat and tell you that you're missing out. Thanksgiving isn't the time to lecture anyone, so it's probably best to just sit there and quietly remember all of the toxins they are taking in their bodies. You might want to warn them, but there's enough drama on Thanksgiving already and we don't need to add to that list.

Even on just regular days, if you are making dinner for someone, or if someone is making dinner for you, you will get the jokes rolling in. "This is good...but it would be even better with meat!" "This is missing something...meat!" Ha, ha, ha. Very funny. You've just got to learn to take it graciously and laugh it off. You can take this as a chance to explain yourself, or just let it roll off your shoulders. It doesn't mean disrespect, really. Some people are just offended that you are choosing a different lifestyle and by doing so, indicating that maybe their lifestyle has something wrong with it.

It's okay to bring your own food. If you are cooking for others, do not lay off the fattening dairy-free butter and oils. You want it to taste as good as possible so that they will see that you are still eating delicious things. If people ask you why you are giving up so much food, simply reply that there are so many foods you can still eat. If they are curious, cook for them or take them to a vegan restaurant and open their eyes! There are literally thousands of different types of fruits and vegetables, and it is highly unlikely that you've tried them all. Vegans that have been eating plant-based for years most likely haven't tried them all! There's always something new to try and different recipes to make, so feel free to reiterate that if someone asks why you are eating "such a restricted" diet.

Some people will even be rude enough to try to slip meat into your diet. While that doesn't happen very often, it can definitely be if your friends are a little feistier. The best way to deal with this is to be firm in your decision and to double-check your meal and under anything that might be hiding meat. If you have any questions about it, ask them. They will most likely fess-up before you eat. Then, be firm in the fact that you will not eat it.

Like I mentioned before, even if you are a laid-back vegan (which most people still think are the best kind), people will notice. You'll be surprised at who decides to support you and maybe even try it with you. You'll also be surprised at what people say to you about it, and about how they admire your dedication. People notice things, whether you want to or not. You might also have to cook a lot more. People tend to become confused on what to make for vegans. They wonder what they could make, and sometimes they are actually scared to even try, because what if they mess it up? Others will think that it's way too much effort to cook for you, which is understandable. Remember what you felt like starting out. It is a little overwhelming at first, and if they have no desire to be vegan, it can seem quite exhausting. If you get invited to dinner, it is always nice to offer to bring a dish, so at least you know you'll have something to eat.

It is hard if someone has cooked something for you and you can't eat it. It can be awkward. Sometimes, it can feel like they think you're attacking them. Just simply explain that you aren't eating dairy or eggs and you are sure it is delicious but personally cannot bring yourself to eat it. Be kind about it, and apologetic, and they can't help but forgive you.

You don't even have to tell people right away, because you might feel like they are judging you or think you are "extreme." Feel free to keep it to yourself until you see the benefits.

Yes, there are awkward situations that you'll have to deal with, but remember how great you'll feel and how amazing you'll look! Don't shy away from these situations, stand your ground instead. It will all turn out okay and you won't regret your decision, especially sticking with it. Remember, you can eat anything you want, you are just choosing not to! You have the power, not anyone else.

Basic Meal Outline

It's probably important to go over the very basics of a vegan diet. The possibilities are endless, as I've said, but it's important to have some kind of guideline. There are many cookbooks out there that give very detailed recipes and how to prepare them. If you're really interested in going vegan, a good cookbook is crucial. My personal favorites are The Happy Herbivore, and Veganomics. There are tons out there that I haven't read, but those have helped me so much going from a vegetarian diet to vegan. There are plenty of specialty vegan cookbooks, as well. You can get some that are all about baking, or you can stick to the ones that specialize in meals that take less time, or meals that are low fat. There are so many different types to go with that the possibilities are endless.

For breakfast, there are many different options. You could make vegan pancakes, tofu scramble, vegan French toast, vegan cinnamon rolls, and a plethora of other options. All of those recipes come up really quick with a web search. The most common vegan breakfasts that are simple and easy, especially good if you are in a hurry, are smoothies and fruit plates. Smoothies can come in a variety of different flavors and types. They can have vegetables, and they can also have fruits and types of seeds in them. An example of a filling smoothie is the chocolate peanut butter banana smoothie. It's delicious, and contains chocolate vegan protein powder, a spoon full of peanut butter, bananas, and some dairy-free milk or water. It's absolutely satisfying and delicious. The fruit platter is probably the simplest type of breakfast. When you eat something as pure and raw as fruit for breakfast, you are setting your entire day up for success.

Next is lunch. If you're bringing lunch to work, it's always simplest to stick with a salad or something that is delicious and easy to prepare. You could also prepare some type of vegan wrap and have avocados, beans, lettuce, spinach, corn, and tomatoes in the wrap. Delicious and easy. Salads can be dressed up and completely different each day. For example, one day you could bring a salad made with spinach and fruit topped with a splash of balsamic vinegar for a sweeter option. The next day, you could create some sort of southwestern salad, with black beans, corn, and tomatoes. It is simple to switch up salads and make them taste exciting. In fact, there is an entire cookbook that has vegan salads you can eat called Salad Samurai. It has 100 different salad recipes! Salads are healthy, filling, and simple, and are some of the best lunches to make. Another easy thing to bring to work is if you make in bulk and warm up. It is easy to cook a one-pot quinoa dish, or something along that sort, and cook a lot of it. If you don't get bored easily, this is a great option, because you can keep bringing it until it's gone. Not much variety, but it is probably the absolute easiest thing to do.

If you have a little more time, you can experiment with lunches and make plenty of things, such as sandwiches on healthy bread with hummus and bean sprouts, loaded oatmeal, big vegetable platters, different types of wraps, or another easy option is to take leftovers from dinner the previous day!

For dinner, it can be the meal with the most variety of them all. This is where it is fun to try different recipes because normally there's a little more time to spare when it comes to cooking dinner. This is the best time to incorporate lots of protein and cook with tofu or tempeh, since it takes such a long time to prepare them. You could make a large burrito bowl, loaded potato (with Earth Balance butter), or have soup in a slow cooker to be ready when you want to eat. You could have Asian-spiced chickpeas, vegan chili, or so many other things. There are so many different options that you will never get bored. The best suggestion is to find new recipes in cookbooks and try them out, if they sound good or not. You'll be surprised at how much you will like out of what you try in the cookbooks.

Always remember the vegan food pyramid while planning meals. Each day, you should aim to have 2-4 servings of vegetables, 1-3 servings of fruit, 3-5 servings of whole grains, 1-2 servings of dairy substitutes, 1-2 servings of beans, legumes, and nuts, and the rest you should use sparingly. If you are a planner, go ahead and plan out the weeks meals and stick to it! Sometimes that is the best way to go. If you aren't, take it a day at a time, and log what you eat in order to see if you are on track. It is important to pay attention to what you are eating because you need to get all the nutrients that lovely body of yours needs to stay healthy. Treat your body right, pay attention to what you are eating, and try to stay within the vegan food pyramid. You'll feel amazing if you follow those guidelines!

Eating vegan doesn't have to mean giving up variety and taste. It can open the doors to variety and taste. Some chefs will swear that they got their love of food from going vegan. It really makes you think outside of the box and opens the door to all types of possibilities.

The Odd Side Effects of Being Vegan

Besides feeling better, which we have discussed in detail, there are other "side effects" of being vegan. You'll feel powerful. You decide what goes in your body, and you have the self-control to actually control what goes into your body. Speaking of your body, after a few months, it will be in the best shape it's ever been in (as long as you eat healthy and exercise, too) and you'll look amazing. You'll feel like a savior because of all of the animals you yourself are singlehandedly saving, and you'll want to shout out to the world how great you feel.

Then, you'll start wondering what other areas of your life you can take control of. If you can make this huge lifestyle change and stick with it, what else can you do? Take this feeling and use it to its full advantage. Go change the things that you have always wondered about. Take control of your body, your life, and everything else that you want to. You're a powerful person, and if you can tackle this, you can do anything you put your mind to.

Maybe you'll ditch the microwave or start adopting a minimalist lifestyle. Maybe you'll run a 5K, 10K, or half marathon. Find something you've wanted to do and just get it done. You can do it, and you will do it.

The most important thing you can take away from this book is that even if you don't completely go for it, at least do it once or twice a week. You'll still notice a difference, and you'll still make a difference. If you are going to go for it, be proud of it. This is a big deal, and a huge lifestyle change. Of course you'll feel the amazing changes, but don't shy away from the reason you have become happier and healthier. Don't let other people's jokes put you down. Know that you are a better you, and be proud of it. You've taken control of your body and what you are putting into it. Be a proud and healthy vegan! Remember the three methods and put them to work. You can do this, and you will be so glad you did.

Good luck, fellow plant-eaters!

www.ingramcontent.com/pod-product-compliance
Lightning Source LLC
Chambersburg PA
CBHW070132290526
45789CB00005B/2212